Food As Medicine: How To Prevent and Cure Diseases Through Food

Henry H Steele

3

DEDICATION

This book is dedicated to my family and friends. They are the most important people in my life, and I love them beyond words.

Table of Contents

ACKNOWLEDGMENTS

"Writing a book is more difficult than I anticipated, but it is also more rewarding than I could have imagined. None of this would have been possible without the trust and belief of my friends and family members in me to complete this wonderful project on the topic **(Food As Medicine: How To Prevent and Cure Diseases Through Food)**, which also assisted me in conducting extensive research and learning about a wide range of topics. They were there for me through every difficulty and every achievement. It is a blessing to be surrounded by such talented and supportive people. Thank you very much. I adore you all."

1.You Are What You Eat

Recent nutritional study has found 14 different nutrient-dense foods that have been shown time and again to enhance good overall health. They are referred to as "superfoods" because they have less calories, higher quantities of vitamins and minerals, and a high concentration of disease-fighting antioxidants.

- Beans (legumes)
- berries (particularly blueberries)
- broccoli
- green tea
- nuts (particularly walnuts)
- oranges
- pumpkin
- and salmon Soy
- spinach
- tomatoes
- turkey
- healthy grains and oats
- and yoghurt

They can all help prevent and even reverse diseases including hypertension, diabetes, Alzheimer's, and certain types of cancer. And, because the entire body is interconnected, what affects one area of the body can also influence the health and functioning of other parts of the body. Weight loss gimmicks and other flyby-night methods might become a thing of the past in your life if you use these 14 foods as the foundation of a balanced, robust diet.

In contrast, the negative effects of an imbalanced diet are numerous and diverse. Low energy levels, mood fluctuations, constant tiredness, weight change, and body discomfort are just a few indicators that your diet is out of balance. An unbalanced diet can lead to concerns with body tissue maintenance, growth and development, brain and neurological system function, and bone and muscular systems.

Malnutrition symptoms include fatigue, irritability, a weakened immune system that leads to frequent colds or allergies, and mineral deficiency, which can lead to a number of health problems, including anemia.

And, because the body and spirit are inextricably linked, it stands to reason that an unhealthy body will result in a sick spirit. When we feed these superfoods to our bodies and supplement them with other nutrient-dense and healthful fresh meals, our spirits will be revitalized and healthy.

Many modern diets centered on pre-packaged convenience meals are deficient in many vitamins and minerals, which can damage our mental capacities and create anger, disorientation, and a constant sense of 'being in a fog. 'Superfoods can form the foundation of a great, healthy, nutritional remedy to many of these problems and other

2. Prevention Is Better Than Cure

Everywhere you look, there's a new drug or prescription that promises to instantly cure your illness, ailment, or health problem. And, while popping a pill to heal whatever ails you may seem easy and straightforward, perhaps it's time to sit down and take a good, long look at what you're feeding your body, or, more accurately, what you're not giving your body. Are you genuinely providing your body with the nutrition it requires to function properly?

When we examine what we've been eating, most of us discover that the decisions we've been making in the name of convenience, simplicity, or saving time have actually been damaging to our total health - body, mind, and spirit.

Our current diet mostly consists of an excess of grain, sugar, fried and fatty foods. As a result, disorders including hypertension, diabetes, obesity, Alzheimer's, and certain malignancies are becoming increasingly widespread.

Healthy foods and nutrition can not only help you stay fit, but they can also assist you treat disease. You might not even need to visit a health food store. You can find them in your local grocery store or at your local farmer's market. Furthermore, the harmful repercussions of these diseases can be mitigated, prevented, or even reversed by focusing on a healthy, well-balanced diet based on the 14 foods.

When you nurture your body physically with these nutrient-dense foods, your mental capacities improve, as does your spiritual welfare. Moreover, because your spiritual health is at its best, it will radiate to the exterior world, causing others to notice you're happier, more relaxed, and your stress levels have decreased dramatically.

So, seek ways to eliminate junk from your diet and replace it with members of the Superfoods group. As a result, your body, mind, and soul will all be healthier.

3. Make Your Way to Daily Health

It is critical that we consume a variety of fruits and vegetables every day. Fruit and vegetable-rich diets may lessen the risk of cancer and other chronic diseases. Fruits and vegetables include necessary vitamins and minerals, fiber, and other compounds that are beneficial to one's health. Most fruits and vegetables are inherently low in fat and calories, and they are satisfying.

You've most likely heard of the 5 A Day for Better Health programmes. It offers simple strategies to incorporate more fruits and veggies into your regular diet. Every day, we must consume a wide array of vibrant orange/yellow, red, green, white, and blue/purple veggies and fruit. You will benefit from the necessary vitamins, minerals, and fiber that each color group has to offer, both alone and in combination, if you consume vegetables and fruit from each colour group.

There are various simple methods to begin introducing veggies and fruit into your regular and favourite meals. You can start your day with 100% fruit or vegetable juice, top your cereal with bananas or strawberries, or have a salad for lunch and an apple for an afternoon snack. With a vegetable for dinner, you've already had around 5 cups of fruits and vegetables. You might also try a piece of fruit as a snack or an additional veggie at supper.

Don't be scared to try something new to enhance your intake of vegetables and fruits. When it comes to fruits and vegetables, there are so many options. Kiwifruit, asparagus, and mango could be your new favourite fruits. Combine fruits and vegetables with contrasting flavours and colours to keep things interesting, such as red grapes with pineapple chunks or cucumbers and red peppers.

Make it a practice to keep fruits and veggies visible and easily available; you'll eat them more. Refrigerate chopped and washed produce at eye level, or keep a large colourful bowl of fruit on the table.

4. To get Your Diet from Healthy Food Is a Lifelong Habit

Many people believe that taking a multivitamin supplement to receive their nutrients is equally as effective as eating whole foods. They are oblivious to the fact that natural foods and beverages are far greater suppliers of vitamins and minerals. Our bodies use vitamins and minerals from whole meals more efficiently. And most people find it far easier to choose a variety of whole foods that they enjoy eating rather than trying to make sense of the vast array of vitamin and mineral supplements available. And anyone who has taken a multivitamin or a mineral supplement will tell you that the taste leaves a lot to be desired.

Supplements are also tough for our systems to digest and utilize, making it challenging to gain the full benefit of the vitamins and minerals they contain. In contrast, eating a lot of nutrient-dense food to acquire the same amount of nutrients means the nutrients will be easier for the body to process and use, and will be less likely to be squandered. When we absorb nutrients via food instead of the 'one a day' approach, we are also processing them throughout the day.

Many supplements on the market now use fillers and binders to keep them together, as well as coatings on the tablets themselves. These are items that the body does not require and will not use. Some people develop allergies to the colours and fillers used in vitamin pills.

The fiber that binds fruits and vegetables, on the other hand, is utilized by the body. The "skin" of a vegetable, such as a potato, is often the most nutritious component. Furthermore, vitamin and mineral supplements might occasionally upset our stomachs, making them even more difficult to take the next day. In many circumstances, mixing supplements might reduce their effectiveness and cause stomach trouble when dealing with the taste and smell of particular vitamins. A variety of fruits and vegetables, on the other hand, enhance the flavour of a nutritious meal while also aiding digestion.

Eating fresh food is essential to a **weight loss plan** if you want to reduce weight. In addition, eating fresh fruits and vegetables keeps hair, skin, and teeth looking and feeling good. And, come to think of it, fruits and vegetables are the original 'To go' food.

It's easy to grab an orange, apple, banana, or grapes, or put a few vegetables together for a quick salad to take to work. So, if you're looking for well-balanced, healthful, and dependable nutrition, avoid the bottle. Go for the food.

5. Weight Loss Foods

Fruits and vegetables, according to experts, are two basic kinds of meals that might be dubbed "keeping it off superfoods" since they fill your tummy without packing on the calories. And what nutrients give fruits and vegetables their staying power?' Fiber. So, if fruits and vegetables are the **"weight-loss food categories**," fiber may be the **"weight-loss super nutrient."** Another super nutrient is protein. Protein is becoming more scientifically recognized as a potential appetite suppressor. Protein also has a long-lasting effect and can somewhat enhance your metabolism. But, as with all things, if you eat more than your body requires, it will show up on the scale as a gain, rather than a loss.

The following foods are low-calorie and healthful solutions that will help you reduce weight:

Green Tea

Researchers believe that the catechins (beneficial phytochemicals) in green tea may help with weight loss by boosting the body's metabolism and moderately decreasing body fat. So, enjoy a hot cup of green tea or a large glass of iced tea.

Soups made with broth or tomatoes

Soups can help reduce appetite before meals and

boost your feeling of fullness.

Green salads with a low-calorie count

As a first dish, having a low-calorie salad – one that isn't heavy with croutons, high-fat dressings, and cheese –will make you feel fuller, allowing you to eat less of your main course. Choose your components well, and its high fiber content could be the key to battling cravings later in the day.

Yogurt

Dairy products will help you lose weight if you include them in your balanced diet. Because of the protein and carbohydrate content, choosing a light yogurt may help you fight off hunger symptoms.

Beans

Beans are a fantastic source of fiber and protein, and they help you feel fuller for longer, which may help you avoid snacking in between meals.

Water

Water is your body's lifeline, and you should drink plenty of it throughout the day. It's a terrific no-calorie beverage that you may get by drinking unsweetened tea, flavoured unsweetened mineral water, normal water with lime or lemon, or even cucumber slices.

It can make you feel full while also flushing toxins from your body. So, the next time you feel hungry, try sipping a glass of water before reaching for a snack.

Whole-Grain Cereal with High Fiber

Whole grains, in general, help to increase the fiber and nutritious worth of your meal. One of the simplest ways to add more whole grains to your diet is to eat a bowl of higher-fiber whole-grain cereal for breakfast or as a snack.

6. Smart Food Choices Can Help You Flush the Fat

Getting rid of the fat? As weird as it may sound, the Fat Flush Plan can help you reshape your body while detoxifying your system. Ann Louise Gittleman, Ph.D., C.N.S. developed this low-carbohydrate, three-phase diet programme.

The plan's first phase, known as The Two-Week Fat Flush, lasts 14 days and is intended to kick-start weight loss.

Phase 2, The Ongoing Fat Flush, assists you in maintaining your weight loss,

Phase 3, The Lifestyle Eating Plan, focuses on long-term weight loss.

The Fat Flush Plan was created to enhance metabolism, flush away bloat, and accelerate the fat-burning process. The commitment to promote a balanced lifestyle and support simple healthy behaviors that appear to have fallen by the wayside in our modern and hectic daily lives is at the heart of the plan. Every component of the plan is geared toward achieving this aim, including beneficial essential fats, protein quantities, antioxidant-rich veggies, modest amounts of fruits, calorie-burning herbs and spices, cleansing diuretic beverages, exercise, journaling, and even sleep.

The Two-Week Fat Flush is designed to jumpstart weight loss with a daily caloric intake of 1,100 to 1,200 calories. It will shape your body by increasing fat loss from your body's main fat storage locations, which are your hips, thighs, and buttocks.

The Ongoing Fat Flush is the next stage for those who need to lose more weight but also prefer to follow a more moderate cleansing programme and have a bit more diversity in their meal choices while still losing weight. With around 1,200 to 1,500 calories per day, this portion of the programme is geared for long-term weight loss. This is the phase you'll be in till you reach your goal weight or size.

The Lifestyle Eating Plan is your long-term weight-control strategy. This phase provides over 1,500 calories each day, giving a fundamental lifelong eating diet meant to boost your vitality and well-being for life.

You can have up to two dairy items and up to two additional friendly carbs. Phase 3 carbohydrates include a wider variety of starchy vegetables and non-gluten hypoallergenic grains. Foods are always introduced one at a time to ensure that no allergic reactions occur and that the meal is properly tolerated by your body.

7. Stress-Relieving Foods

Some days, life has a way of getting the best of us. Working too many hours, relocating your children for activities, caring for your household, or dealing with personal or family concerns can all lead to stress, which can be physically, psychologically, emotionally, and spiritually draining. There are, however, basic steps you may take to counteract stress, beginning with the foods you eat.

When life is exceptionally stressful, avoiding caffeine and alcohol is an excellent place to start. Stimulants and depressants like these can drain your vitality and deprive you of the fuel you need to deal with stress. Sugary foods should also be avoided since they cause your blood sugar levels to jump and then drop rapidly, causing your energy levels to spike and drop at the same rate. However, there are a number of superfoods available that will supply you with the energy and nourishment your body requires to keep stress at check. Some are as follows: -

Asparagus

It has a lot of folic acid; it can help you feel better. Folic acid and vitamin B are important in the production of serotonin, a neurotransmitter that makes you happy.

Red Meat

And, despite what we hear about red meat, it's actually a good supper option for a stressed-out family. Beef's high quantities of iron, zinc, and B vitamins not only help you get into a happy mood, but also keep you there. Your butcher can assist you in selecting lean cuts for the healthiest selections.

Milk

Milk is extremely beneficial to one's health. It helps build bones and supports healthy cell regeneration since it is high in calcium, protein, antioxidants, and vitamins B2 and B12. Low-fat milk, paired with a healthy whole-grain cereal choice in the morning, is a terrific way to start your day and prepare yourself to face the pressures that await you. Cottage cheese is another excellent dairy option, and when combined with a vitamin C-rich fruit, it aids the body in combating free radicals that proliferate during stressful times.

Almonds

When it comes to stress relief, almonds are also an excellent choice. They're strong in magnesium, zinc, vitamins B2, C, and E, and unsaturated fats, all of which are powerful antioxidants that fight free radicals, which have been linked to cancer and heart disease.

8.Brain-Boosting Foods

We've all experienced days when we didn't feel 'on our game.' And as we become older, both our bodies and our brains get older. However, by adopting wise eating choices, we may extend the life of our important grey matter and boost brain function. Here are some clever options for maintaining our brains in tip-top form.

Blueberries

They have been found in studies to protect the brain against stress, dementia, and Alzheimer's disease. Blueberry-rich diets have also been demonstrated to boost both learning capacity and motor skills in studies.

Avocados

Although being classified as a "fatty fruit," helps to improve blood flow and lower blood pressure, lowering the risk of developing hypertension, which can lead to a stroke.

Salmon

Deep-water fish is a wise freshwater fish pick. It's high in omega-3 essential fatty acids, which are necessary for proper brain function.

Nuts and seeds

They are high in vitamin E, a nutrient that your brain requires to maintain cognitive function. Almonds, cashews, peanuts, walnuts, sunflower and sesame seeds, and cashews are all excellent alternatives.
Other than the food mentioned above following food also help to maintain a healthy brain

- Whole-grain breads
- brown rice
- oatmeal

They help by lowering the risk of cardiovascular disease. The brain will thrive due to great oxygen and nutrition delivery through the bloodstream if a healthy heart and enhanced blood flow are promoted.

Complex carbs

They also provide the brain with a continuous supply of glucose, which improves brain function. Simple carbohydrates, such as those found in junk food, should be avoided since they provide the brain with a short-term sugar high, followed by a fall that makes you feel hungry and exhausted.

Freshly brewed tea (black tea)

It also contains strong antioxidants, particularly the catechins class, which supports healthy blood flow. Because black tea contains caffeine, it is vital to use it responsibly.

Dark chocolate

They include potent antioxidants, many natural stimulants that boost focus and concentration, and it promotes the creation of endorphins, which helps improve mood. Again, moderation is essential.

9.Body, Mind, and Spirit Rejuvenation Foods

When the goal is to rejuvenate the body, mind, and spirit, smaller, more frequent snacks and meals should be used. This will help you maintain a consistent energy level and manage your blood sugar levels to minimize spikes and troughs. When you choose the perfect balance of foods, your body receives the much-needed boost it needs to sustain itself effectively, even during those afternoon slumps. So, instead of reaching for high-sugar junk meals, try the following to get the boost you need.

Any fresh fruit, especially those with skins or seeds, such as **peaches, apples, pears, oranges, and strawberries,** is high in vitamins and fiber. In the summer, a peach provides plenty of dietary fiber, niacin (vitamin B3), potassium, beta carotene, and vitamin A, as well as significant levels of vitamin C. Niacin is essential for supplying energy for cell tissue formation. Along with controlling fluid balance, potassium contributes to the electrical stability of your heart and nervous system cells and is necessary for cell and muscle growth. Vitamin B12 aids in the development of red blood cells, neurological function, and the metabolism of protein and fat.

The combination of **dried apricots** and **almonds** has a lot of vitamin A, iron, protein, and fiber. Both foods are low in cholesterol and sodium, and apricots are high in potassium, which helps regulate your body's fluid balance. Apricots include vitamin A, which promotes good vision, bone growth, and reproduction, as well as aiding in the fight against infection.

Raisins are a low-fat, low-cholesterol, and low-sodium snack that contain significant amounts of potassium, phosphorus, copper, and iron, as well as riboflavin (vitamin B2) and vitamin B12, as well as a high amount of calcium, which is required not only for strong bones and teeth but also for the normal functioning of the heart and other muscles when combined with low-fat yoghurt.

Beta carotene, vitamin A, vitamin C, folate, vitamin B6, iron, potassium, copper, and fiber are all found in small amounts in **baby carrots** and **sesame sticks**. Beta carotene aids in the prevention of diseases such as heart disease and cancer.

Vitamin A is necessary for healthy skin, improved night vision, and the prevention of infection and respiratory illnesses. Folate, also known as vitamin B9, is necessary for human survival, as it aids in the formation of red blood cells, the breakdown of proteins, and cell growth and division.

Peanut butter on whole grain crackers is a high-protein, iron, niacin, and fiber source. Peanut butter on celery is a classic snack that stays fresh for a long time, and celery is high in vitamins, minerals, and fiber. Low-fat string cheese is a fantastic source of calcium and protein in a hurry. They come in individual servings that are convenient to transport, and you can add a piece of fresh fruit for added fiber.

10.Heartburn-Relieving Foods

Millions of individuals suffer from heartburn and indigestion. Consistent digestive issues can be a sign of overeating, poor dietary habits, or something more serious. Simple dietary modifications, on the other hand, can bring relief.

Several meals can cause heartburn or indigestion by relaxing the band of muscles at the end of your oesophagus, allowing stomach acid to pass through. Heartburn and indigestion can be considerably reduced or avoided by avoiding spicy foods with **black pepper or chili powder, garlic and raw onions, citrus foods like tomatoes, oranges, and grapefruit, fried or fatty foods, alcohol** or anything with **caffeine such as coffee, tea, or soft drinks.**

Make sure you consume plenty of fiber from a range of veggies, non-citrus fruits, and whole grains for overall healthy digestion and to reduce acid reflux. Drink enough water to help your body absorb critical nutrients and decrease food waste, and cook with low-fat ingredients. After supper or before night, try sipping herbal chamomile tea, which is thought to have a relaxing effect on the stomach.

Heartburn and indigestion episodes can be reduced by eating smaller, more frequent meals. Make sure you eat your meals and snacks in a quiet, relaxing environment with little to no noise or interruptions.

Wear loose-fitting clothing that isn't too tight around the waist and abdomen, and don't lie down just after a meal.

Make **oatmeal** for breakfast. It's high in fiber, low in saturated fat and cholesterol, and gives you a calcium boost when paired with skim milk. If you add blueberries or raisins to the mix, you'll get some extra iron and potassium for a well-balanced dinner.

If you're looking for a lean, nutrient-dense protein source that's also easy on the stomach, turkey is the way to go. **Turkey** is abundant in niacin, a B vitamin that helps decrease blood cholesterol levels. Chicken without the skin is also a good low-fat protein source. Both are simple to prepare, whether inside or outside.

Apples and grapes are low in saturated fat, cholesterol, and salt, and are a good source of vitamin C and fiber in a non-citrus fruit.

11.Cold-Relieving Foods

Healthy, nutrient-dense foods not only nourish your body and aid in cell growth and reproduction, but they also help arm your body's defenses against bacteria that cause colds. Low-fat meats, whole grains, fruits, veggies, and whole grains all contribute to your body's readiness for fight.

Water is another vital component of your anti-cold defence mechanism. When you're dehydrated, your body is more vulnerable to viruses latching on and refusing to let go. Drink plenty of water and decaffeinated beverages to keep your body hydrated and ready.

One cup of **yogurt** each day may help keep the gastrointestinal tract healthy, which can help prevent colds. It must be yogurt with live cultures, as this is the crucial element that keeps the GI tract in good working order. And there's an added benefit to eating yogurt: recent research suggests that eating dairy on a daily basis can help you lose weight or maintain a healthy weight.

Garlic contains allicin, an antibiotic that has been demonstrated in certain studies to prevent cold complications. Garlic may be added to many of your favourite foods to enhance flavour and help you prepare for the fight against cold germs.

An **apple** a day keeps the doctor away, so the saying goes. So can an orange. One orange per day delivers your recommended daily amount of vitamin C. Oranges are also high in flavonoids, which help your body's cells repair and stay healthy and robust.

Green bell peppers are the best source of vitamin C in the vegetable family. Add them to a salad or just eat them raw. Flavonoids can also be present in peppers. You could even make a green pepper dip seasoned with garlic for increased germ-fighting power.

Lean ground beef, especially when cooked with garlic, can help to preserve cell health and fight off sickness. It's high in protein, selenium, and zinc, and when combined with a little of tomato, it's an excellent cold-weather food.

12. Flu-Fighting Foods

Flu outbreaks account for millions of wasted hours at work and home each year, not to mention countless terrible days spent trying to recover. If you're wondering what you can do to naturally boost your immunity and prepare your body's defenses, look at the foods you're eating, as well as the meals your family is eating, and make the necessary changes to ensure everyone is eating a well-balanced diet rich in nutrient-dense fruits and vegetables, low-fat proteins, and complex carbohydrates.

Black currants contain nearly three times the recommended daily consumption for adults, making them even more vitamin C-rich than oranges. It is critical to consume adequate amounts of vitamin C since it aids in the prevention of infections and the maintenance of a healthy immune system.

Replace **orange juice** in your morning breakfast with grapefruit juice for a vitamin C-rich drink that's both sweet and tangy. However, if you are taking medications for high blood pressure, AIDS, anxiety, or hay fever, you should consult your doctor first, as grapefruit juice can cause serious toxicity when combined with certain medications.

Brussel sprouts are an excellent source of vitamin C, are strong in fiber, and are high in folate. They enhance the anticarcinogenic capabilities of glycosylated, which are key cancer-fighting compounds. They're a terrific way to add a lot of flu-busting nutrients to a stew.

Yogurt with living cultures has a favourable effect on your GI tract, which helps the body eliminate germs from the body more rapidly and effectively, as well as fight the flu. You want your yoghurt to include the active culture L. acidophilus, which aids in the battle against yeast infections.

Potatoes are one of the most economical sources of vitamin C, and their high levels of potassium and fiber enhance any entrée wonderfully. The skin has the greatest fiber, but the flesh directly beneath the surface has the most vitamin C. The finest source of vitamin C is fresh potatoes. Be mindful of how you prepare them, as soaking them in water depletes them of their germ-fighting vitamin C.

Whole wheat pasta is also high in niacin, fiber, and iron. Its complex carbohydrates are an important part of a healthy diet that will keep your immune system strong. Simply replace regular spaghetti in recipes with whole wheat pasta for a delicious and healthful spin on your favourite pasta meals.

13.Foods for Strong Bones

Many people believe that the primary cause of osteoporosis is a lack of calcium in their diet. However, calcium is only a minor component of the entire picture. While calcium supplements can be beneficial, there are other nutritional issues to consider.

In fact, the primary dietary cause of osteoporosis is the use of extremely acidic foods such as refined white sugar, refined white flour, high-fructose corn syrup, soft drinks, cookies, candies, sweets, desserts, and anything containing sweeteners.

When these goods are consumed in excess, the pH level in your blood becomes extremely acidic. To counteract this, your body seeks for calcium and magnesium and releases it into your bloodstream in an attempt to maintain a healthy pH level.

As a result, every soft drink, candy, cake, and treat you consume depletes the bone density of your skeleton. The calcium and magnesium that your body gathers in an attempt to offset this acidic environment is transferred through your kidneys, where it might contribute to kidney stones, and then departs your body through your urine.

Simply avoid consuming any white flour, processed sugars, added sugars, soft drinks, sweets, candies, breads, or any other items created with refined carbohydrates to avoid losing bone mass.

Furthermore, nutrients such as **broccoli, cabbage, celery**, and other **dark green leafy vegetables** assist maintain a good pH balance. Calcium and magnesium must be obtained from healthy sources, such as organic, plant-based vitamins. You should also boost your diet with sea vegetables, which are naturally alkaline. These include seaweed, kelp, and a variety of others. **Sprouts** are another fantastic food option.

14. Heart-healthy Foods

In the United States, heart disease is the top cause of death for both men and women. And, while we are all aware that consuming nutrient-dense healthy foods helps minimize the risk, we may not be aware of which foods are the greatest alternatives for combating this terrible disease.

The idea is to increase fiber and choose unsaturated fats. Unsaturated fats, such as omega-3 fatty acids and olive oil, can help lower triglycerides. A diet high in soluble fiber, which is commonly found in legumes and other fruits and vegetables, also aids in the reduction of LDL cholesterol levels.

Sardines are high in omega-3 fatty acids, as well as calcium and niacin. You can grill fresh sardines, or use canned sardines in salads or sandwiches. **Mackerel** is another high-quality source of omega-3 fatty acids, as well as a good amount of selenium, an antioxidant mineral that may help protect the body from heart disease and cancer. A handful of **walnuts** for an afternoon snack is a fantastic way to obtain omega-3s on the road. Add some to your green salad, or add ground walnuts to your chicken salad for a nutritional boost.

Kidney beans are an inexpensive source of high fiber, low fat, and cholesterol-free. They're great in salads and chili, and they're almost a perfect healthy food. Because canned kinds are higher in salt, utilize dried ones whenever feasible.

Whole-grain barley is high in soluble and insoluble fiber, which helps with constipation. It's also high in iron and minerals and a rich source of protein. Choose whole-grain barley cereals or replace rice and pasta side dishes with whole-grain barley once a week.

Oatmeal is a fantastic method to increase your fiber level in the morning, and it also has a low glycaemic index, which helps to deliver lasting energy and fight off hunger. Choose rolled oats and season with raisins, apples, and honey. Instant oatmeal isn't a healthy option because it's usually filled with sugar.

15. Cancer-Fighting Foods

Cancer is the second most lethal disease in the United States, and it comes with a slew of risk factors. As a result, it's only natural that we look at our diets and start including nutrient-dense foods that have been found to reduce cancer risk. A diet high in fiber, vegetables, and fruits, as well as liquids produced entirely from fruit juice, can significantly reduce your cancer risk.

Beans and phytochemical-rich cruciferous vegetables such as broccoli, cauliflower, cabbage, brussels sprouts, and kale are suitable substitutes. Dark green leafy vegetables such as spinach, romaine lettuce, and collard greens are also high in fiber, lutein, and carotenoids, all of which are cancer-fighting compounds. Choose foods rich in vitamins C, E, and A, all of which are antioxidants in and of themselves. These help to limit the formation of free radicals in your body, which helps to protect you against cancer.

Tomatoes are a fantastic anti-cancer superfood. Tomatoes are strong in lycopene, an antioxidant phytochemical that also aids in the prevention of heart disease, as well as vitamins A, C, and E, all of which aid in the battle against cancer-causing free radicals. Toss them in a salad or use them as a topping for homemade pizza. They're also a tasty way to spruce up your favourite sandwich.

Watermelon is particularly high in antioxidants and contains almost 80% of your daily vitamin C intake. It's also high in beta carotene, a type of vitamin A. It also contains lycopene, which is found in tomatoes.

Cabbage is a cruciferous vegetable that aids in the prevention of colon and rectal cancers. Cabbage is also high in fiber and contains over half of the daily vitamin C requirement, making it a well-rounded food with cancer-fighting properties. Carrots are also high in fiber and beta carotene, and they contain nearly three times the daily vitamin A needed.

Did you know that a quarter cup of **kidney beans** equals two ounces of red meat in terms of fiber and protein? Whole wheat pasta is particularly high in fiber, and broccoli will help you meet your daily vitamin A and C requirements. Toss them all together with your favourite low-fat Italian dressing for a quick and easy dinner that will help you fight cancer.

Strawberries and **blueberries** are high in vitamin C and fiber. They're a quick and easy finger food that goes well with whole grain cereal, oatmeal, or low-fat yoghurt.

16. Foods to Help You Beat Arthritis Pain

It's simple to incorporate these nutrient-dense foods into your daily diet with a little thought and planning. With options from nearly every food group, you'll soon be well on your way to arming yourself to battle arthritis pain and begin to manage it from the inside out.

Salmon is high in healthful fats, making it an excellent source of omega-3 fatty acids. Salmon is also high in calcium, vitamin D, and folate. Salmon may protect the cardiovascular system by preventing blood clots, mending arterial damage, increasing good cholesterol levels, and reducing blood pressure, in addition to aiding with arthritis.

Bananas, often referred to as one of nature's "perfect foods," are high in potassium, but they're also high in arthritis-fighting vitamin B6, folate, and vitamin C. They're easy for your body to digest, and because they're high in soluble fiber, they're a crucial player in your weight loss efforts because they make you feel full without consuming a lot of calories.

If you're looking for vitamin C but don't like citrus fruits, try a **green pepper**. A single green pepper provides 176 percent of your daily vitamin C requirements, and vibrant red and yellow types provide more than double that amount. Sweet peppers are higher in vitamin C than citrus fruits, but they are also high in vitamin B6 and folate.

Vitamin D is difficult to find in foods, but shrimp fits the bill, with around 30% of the daily necessary amount in about three ounces — significantly more than a cup of milk. **Shrimp** also contains omega-3 fatty acids and vitamin C, as well as other elements important for overall health, such as iron and vitamin B12.

Cheese, whether hard or soft, fresh or ripened, is a wonderful source of calcium for bones and protein for muscles and other joint-supporting tissues. Cheese can be sliced to go on a cracker or sandwich, grated into your favourite recipe, or eaten with an apple or pear for a fresh, quick snack.

Green tea includes hundreds of potent antioxidant compounds known as polyphenols, which have been linked to a lower risk of cancer and heart disease. However, research suggests that green tea may help prevent or alleviate the symptoms of rheumatoid arthritis.

17. Alzheimer's Disease-Fighting Foods

Alzheimer's disease is a degenerative brain ailment that eventually damages memory as well as thinking and reasoning abilities. According to recent estimates, around 4 million people in the United States have dementia, the majority of whom have Alzheimer's disease. By 2050, that figure might rise to 16 million.

However, by making a few simple changes to your diet to incorporate more folate-rich foods, you can help minimize your risk. According to studies, older persons whose diets were high in folate cut their risk of Alzheimer's disease in half when compared to those whose diets contained less than the RDA.

Folate has also been proven to lower homocysteine levels in the blood, which is a risk factor for heart disease. High levels of homocysteine, as well as low levels of folate and vitamin B-12, have also been linked to stroke and Alzheimer's disease.

A healthy, well-balanced diet is your best bet for getting enough folate. Make sure you consume at least five servings of fresh fruits and vegetables every day. **Oranges and bananas, dark leafy green vegetables, asparagus, broccoli, liver,** and many varieties of **beans and peas,** including **lima, lentil,** and **garbanzo,** as well as **fortified breads** and **cereals**, are high in folate.

Apple antioxidants may help protect the brain from the type of damage that underlies Alzheimer's and Parkinson's disease, according to new research. However, it is estimated that the average American consumes only one-seventh of an apple each day, which is far from adequate.

Blueberries are also an excellent food choice for arming your body against deteriorating mental capacities. It's also critical to choose unsaturated fats to keep your circulatory system healthy. Healthy blood flow and blood arteries reduce the risk of brain damage caused by strokes or poor circulation.

18. Foods For a Long and Healthy Life

According to new research, certain chemicals in foods, such as sulforaphane, a phytochemical found in broccoli, work with your genes to boost your body's natural defence systems, helping in the inactivation of toxins and free radicals before they cause cancer, heart disease, and even premature ageing.

And the objective for the future is to be able to predict which diseases or maladies someone is genetically predisposed to so that their diets can be tailored properly. We'll know which ones to add and which to avoid, and we'll be able to take proactive steps to prevent or repel hereditary diseases. Meanwhile, many foods have been discovered to have anti-aging benefits.

Lycopene, a red pigment found in **tomatoes**, appears to reduce the incidence of heart disease, cancer, and macular degeneration. It's also linked to an increase in geriatric self-sufficiency. While fresh tomatoes are high in lycopene, the most absorbable forms are found in cooked tomato products such as spaghetti sauce and soup, as well as prepared salsas. Pink grapefruit, guava, red bell peppers, and watermelon all contain lycopene.

At least two cups of **orange fruits**, such as **sweet potatoes, squash,** and **carrots,** boost beta-carotene intake, which converts to vitamin A, which is needed for healthy skin and eyes and may also help to prevent cancer, cardiovascular disease, and osteoporosis. Oranges contain the antioxidants lutein and lycopene, which can help prevent macular degeneration, protect skin from UV damage, and even reduce wrinkles. Beta-carotene is abundant in mangoes and cantaloupes.

Eat your **dark leafy greens** if you don't do anything else to change your diet. They've been proven to reduce the risk of heart disease and may even save your sight. Dietary standards require at least three cups of greens each week. Fresh is just as good as frozen or packaged food.

Don't overlook the mental ageing process. Omega 3 fatty acids, which are beneficial to the heart, have also been discovered to help keep your mind sharp. A recent study found that consuming more fatty fish reduces the incidence of mental decline. If fresh fish isn't available, **canned tuna, salmon**, and **sardines** work well.

19. Hair-Healthy Foods

We've all learnt over time that eating a well-balanced diet is beneficial to our bodies and necessary for optimal health and performance. Our hair is no exception. For healthy, strong hair, a combination of protein, complex carbs, vitamins, minerals, and iron is essential.

The first step toward excellent hair nutrition is to have enough protein, which is the building block of your hair. Then you'll need complex carbohydrates to help with protein synthesis, which is necessary for hair growth. B complex, which is linked to energy production and the development of healthy hair and skin, folic acid, B12, and zinc are all crucial vitamins and minerals.

Hair follicles, like us, may have low levels of energy. As a result, it's critical that you have a high-protein meal first thing in the morning. To help your hair grow and thrive in the healthiest way possible, consider the following breakfast and other daily meal selections.

Try eating **red meat** twice a week if you don't have high cholesterol. It contains the protein your hair requires, as well as B vitamins, iron, and zinc, all of which are essential for healthy hair. Bacon is also a good choice because it's high in B vitamins, zinc, and protein, but it's also heavy in calories, so it's not ideal for weight loss.

Eggs and **egg whites** are another great source of protein, especially for vegetarians or those who can't eat red meat or bacon due to dietary constraints. Salmon is another excellent protein option for breakfast, lunch, or dinner. It also contains a lot of B vitamins, including B12, as well as a lot of other vitamins and minerals.

Just keep in mind that, in addition to protein, you should consume complex carbohydrates, which offer energy for a longer period of time than processed carbohydrates. Brown short-grain rice is the best option. It also contains some fiber and is a rich source of B vitamins. Whole grain options supplement your protein intake by assisting in the organization of proteins for optimal hair development and health.

20. Anti-Depression Foods

We've all been down in the dumps at some point in our lives. When they happen on a regular basis, though, it becomes a matter for concern. There are, however, ways to alter your diet to help you maintain a more stable mood. Consume meals at regular intervals to maintain your serotonin levels. Serotonin is a neurotransmitter in the brain with a calming effect. The best defence against depression is a good diet.

Carbohydrates are linked to the production of serotonin, therefore a lack of them can have an effect on your mood. Here are some more food ideas to help you overcome sadness and get rid of the blues.

Dinners that are high in omega-3 fatty acids, such as **salmon** and **mackerel**, are always a wonderful choice. Omega-3 fatty acids also aid in the prevention of heart disease and stroke, as well as several malignancies. Salmon also contains a lot of selenium, which is an antioxidant mineral. Choose wild salmon over farmed or Atlantic salmon at the grocery store or local fish market since it has more omegas.

A recent study found that people suffering from depression had lower levels of the antioxidant vitamin E. Canola oil is high in vitamin E despite being heavy in fat and should be used in moderation. Sautéing meals and veggies with it is a healthier option.

Folate, a vital participant in the creation of serotonin, is abundant in dark green vegetables like **spinach** and **peas**. They are also high in fiber and vitamin C. Fresh is always preferable to canned, as canned foods have a lower nutritional value. Legumes are high in folate, protein, and low in fat, making them a wonderful choice for vegetarians and those who avoid meat.

Chickpeas are high in fiber, iron, and vitamin E. In a blender or food processor, combine a can of drained and rinsed chickpeas, minced garlic, fresh lemon juice, and olive or canola oil for a quick snack. Season to taste with salt, pepper, and other spices. The hummus that results is a nutritious and filling veggie dip.

Both chicken and turkey are high in vitamin B6, which aids in the generation of serotonin in the body.

Selenium, as well as other vitamins and minerals, are abundant in both.

49

If you've had depression symptoms for a long period, see your doctor to discuss therapy options and medications that may be available to you.

<u>21. Sex-Boosting Foods</u>

Every component of a cuisine — its colour, shape, scent, and texture – has the potential to make it sexy. Furthermore, several meals include chemicals that make us feel good by interacting with our hormones or stimulating our brain. Consider implementing some of the following into your next candlelit meal to help you and your companion relax.

Oysters are high in protein and high in minerals such as selenium and zinc. A gorgeous appetizer to a beautiful meal – but be cautious when purchasing, since some may contain high amounts of contaminants like PCB. Oysters should be avoided if you are pregnant.

Chocolate has been a symbol of love and lust for generations due to theobromine, a brain stimulant that produces a pleasurable feeling. Chocolate also includes antioxidants, which may lessen the risk of cancer and heart disease. However, chocolate is heavy in fat, therefore moderation is required. Dark chocolates are often lower in sugar but higher in antioxidants and theobromine than milk chocolate.

Kiwi and **papaya** are vibrant fruits with an enticing and intriguing element that can assist flip the switch. Tropical fruits are high in antioxidants and can help prevent heart disease and cancer. Kiwi contains more vitamin C than an orange, and papaya is abundant in beta-carotene and fiber.

In mediaeval times, mixing **honey** into a drink was thought to sweeten the marriage. However, keep in mind that it still contains a lot of sugar, so take it with caution.

Asparagus might also assist to put your companion in a good mood. It is a natural diuretic and one of the few decent sources of vitamin E. The best way to prepare them without losing nutrients is to steam them, and they can be eaten by hand.

After that romantic supper, a decent cup of coffee or tea boosts the release of adrenaline, which contributes to physical stimulation. It is also present in dark chocolate. Just don't drink too much coffee before bedtime unless you want to be awake all night.

22. Foods To Aid In Menstrual Management

It's the same thing every month. You're bloated, fatigued, and angry, and you're fighting urges and trying to avoid headaches. You wish you could be like your friend or sibling, who seems to breeze through her period with little to no difficulty. Examine your diet to check if these foods are present. If they aren't, they can easily become a part of a well-balanced healthy diet, making your cycles easier to control.

Bananas have long been regarded as the most nutritious food of nature. They include a lot of potassium, zinc, iron, folic acid, calcium, B6, and fiber. They're beneficial for digestion, menstruation problems, and athletes since they can swiftly replenish what your body loses during your period or when you exercise frequently. If you suffer diarrhea during your monthly cycle, combine them with apples, rice, and dry toast, sometimes known as the BRAT therapy.

Famous athletes who consume bee pollen on a regular basis for strength and endurance have popularized it.

It has been used successfully to treat allergies, asthma, menstruation irregularities, constipation, diarrhea, anemia, poor energy, cancer, rheumatism, arthritis, and toxic diseases. It can, however, cause allergic reactions in those who are taking it for the first time, so start with little quantities and gradually increase to a teaspoon or two every day. Bee pollen can be consumed as a powder, capsule, or tablet, or as raw unprocessed honey mixed with porridge or spread on toast.

Make sure you're eating plenty of iron-rich foods. **Green leafy vegetables, beans, seafood, red meat, poultry, and soy foods** are all excellent choices. Combine them with citrus foods high in vitamin C, which will aid in iron absorption. Avoid alcoholic beverages, caffeinated beverages, and salty foods, and always choose unsaturated fats. These would just aggravate the bloated sensation you have every month.

23. Menopause Foods

Including these foods in your diet will help relieve menopausal symptoms, retain memory function, and prevent osteoporosis. These foods are delightful to eat, simple to prepare, and extremely beneficial to your health!

Tofu is a plant-based protein that can be used In place of meat. Tofu, like other soy products, can help you lower your cholesterol and prevent heart disease. Soy products, such as tofu, may also help to reduce the adverse symptoms of menopause, such as the dreaded 'hot flashes.'

Navy beans are high in fiber, which can help reduce your risk of colorectal and other cancers, as well as relieve the symptoms of diverticulosis. Women require 30 grams of fiber per day, so use them in your favourite chili recipe or as a side dish alternative to pasta or rice.

Yogurt, which is high in calcium, can help prevent

osteoporosis. It has also been proved to increase immunity and aid in weight loss. Yogurt also contains a lot of healthy bacteria, such acidophilus, which helps to prevent yeast infections and urinary tract infections. It also contains protein, which may help your body deal with the lethargy and weariness that comes after a hot flash.

We occasionally forget things or feel as though we're in a fog as we become older. If this is the case, pick up some blueberries the next time you go grocery shopping. According to recent research, they may potentially help with short-term memory loss. They're also high in antioxidants. Combine them with low-fat plain yoghurt for an excellent approach to protect both your brain and your bones.

Avocado also includes antioxidants like vitamin E, which can help protect your vision and skin, both of which can deteriorate as we age. Avocados' monounsaturated fat has also been proved to benefit the quality of hair and skin. They're delicious on a turkey sandwich, or mash up a few ripe ones and make a quick side of guacamole to serve with low-fat baked tortilla chips.

And, as usual, when meal planning, make low-fat and low-sodium selections. These are harmful decisions at any age, but especially as we get older, and do little to assist reduce the symptoms of menopause. Avoiding smoking and alcohol, as well as getting plenty of rest, will help you manage your menopause symptoms quickly.

Foods for a Smooth Menopause Transition:

For many women, menopause is a difficult transition. It usually starts in late middle age, when the ovaries' effectiveness begins to wane. Arteriosclerosis, osteoporosis, decreased skin elasticity, and alterations in the sympathetic nerve system that result in "hot flashes" are all problems connected with oestrogen insufficiency. However, by integrating the following foods in your daily diet, you can reduce symptoms, retain memory function, and avoid osteoporosis.

Tofu is a great protein substitute for meat, and it can help you lower your cholesterol and prevent heart disease. Tofu and other soy products may also help reduce menopausal symptoms such as hot flashes.

Fiber has been found in recent research to help reduce the chance of colon and other types of cancer, as well as diverticulosis. Every day, women require roughly 30 grams of fiber. Navy beans weigh 19 grams, making them an excellent choice. Use them in chili or soups, or serve them as a healthful side dish instead of pasta or rice.

As we become older, we may notice that our memory begins to deteriorate and we begin to forget things. We may be able to prevent short-term memory loss by eating blueberries. Toss them on top of plain yoghurt for a delicious breakfast or snack. Yogurt, which is high in calcium, can help in the prevention of osteoporosis. As an added benefit, it can help boost your immunity and aid in your weight loss attempts. Choose yoghurts that are high in probiotics, such as acidophilus, which can help prevent yeast and urinary tract infections.

Avocados are abundant in antioxidants like vitamin E, which is essential for safeguarding your vision and skin. They also contain monosaturated fats, which have been demonstrated to help the quality of a woman's hair and skin, which can suffer during menopause. Cut up a ripe avocado for a tasty guacamole dip, or put it on your sandwich with a tomato.

Avoid drinking a lot of caffeinated drinks every day, and pair an orange with an iron-rich item like whole-grain oatmeal to enhance your body's vitamin C absorption.

24. Healthy Prostate Foods

The prostate gland has a bad reputation for wreaking havoc on one's health. The urethra is strangled by prostate hypertrophy, which affects practically every senior male. This inconvenient condition makes urination difficult and raises the risk of bladder infections and kidney damage. However, there are numerous foods that you may already be eating that can help prevent the start of prostate problems.

Lycopene, a plant pigment known for its cancer-fighting effects, is abundant in **tomatoes, watermelons, red grapefruit, papaya,** and **red berries**. It also helps men maintain prostate health by promoting a robust immune system. Though fresh tomatoes are always a wonderful choice, the lycopene in cooked tomatoes is easier to absorb. It is also an ally in the fight against heart disease.

Quercetin, a flavonoid that serves as the foundation for many other flavonoids, may have beneficial effects in treating or preventing many different types of cancer, including prostate cancer. It also acts as an antihistamine and has anti-inflammatory qualities, which may aid in the relief of pain caused by an inflamed prostate.

Quercetin is abundant in **apples, black and green tea, onions, raspberries, red grapes, citrus fruits, broccoli** and other leafy green vegetables, and cherries. Quercetin can also be found in **honey** and sap, such as that produced by eucalyptus and tea tree blooms.

It's crucial to remember to eat a healthy balance of foods, including antioxidants and vitamin E from nuts and seeds, as well as drink enough of clear fluids to help flush the bladder. Avoid caffeinated beverages, alcoholic beverages, and spicy foods. Maintaining a healthy weight will also help you keep a healthy prostate.

25. Erectile Dysfunction Foods

Erectile dysfunction can be caused by a variety of physical and psychological factors. The most common physical causes are reduced blood flow to the penis and nerve damage. Underlying diseases related with erectile dysfunction include vascular illness, diabetes, medications, hormone abnormalities, neurological disorders, pelvic trauma, surgery, radiation therapy, a venous leak, or psychological concerns.

Zinc deficiency can interfere with the maturation of reproductive organs as well as reproductive activities and processes. It has the potential to contribute to impotence. Chronic diarrhea, weak appetite, and thus severe weight loss of the harmful and unwanted kind, hair loss, and sluggish wound healing are all symptoms of zinc deficiency. Open sores on the skin and in the mouth, unusual tastes in the tongue, and inefficient or impaired mental functioning, particularly cognitive activities, are all symptoms. So, make sure to eat enough zinc-rich foods, such as **red meat, fortified cereals, oysters, almonds, peanuts, chickpeas, soy foods**, and **dairy goods.**

Zinc is essential for many bodily activities, including immunological function, reproduction, and nervous system function.

Other vitamins and minerals should also be included in your diet because they may assist improve erectile dysfunction. Consume foods that are entire, fresh, unrefined, and unprocessed. Include **fruits** (especially plenty of strongly coloured berries to maintain vascular integrity), **vegetables, whole grains, soy, beans, seeds, nuts, olive oil, and cold-water fish** (salmon, tuna, sardines, halibut, and mackerel). Sugar, dairy products, processed foods, fried foods, junk foods, and caffeine should all be avoided.

If you've discovered that you're sensitive to particular foods in the past, eliminate them from your diet since they may be a contributing factor to erectile dysfunction. Make sure to drink plenty of water as well. A good rule of thumb is to drink half your body weight in ounces of water per day (e.g., if you weigh 150 lbs, drink 75 oz of water daily). Avoiding alcohol and smoking might have a negative impact on erectile function.

Erectile dysfunction can be chronic or recurring, or it

might arise as a one-time occurrence. Previously, it was considered that impotence was purely a psychological issue, but many therapists and physicians now feel that the majority of cases of impotence had some physical basis.

<u>26. Natural And Healthy Conception with Foods</u>

For conception and pregnancy to occur, the hormone balance in both the female and male bodies must be just right. Nutrient excess or shortage can upset the balance and disrupt the pregnancy process. When we eat whole meals, we boost our chances of acquiring all of the nutrients we need.

Whole foods include fruits, vegetables, unprocessed **grains, beans, nuts, seeds, eggs,** and **small whole fish**. It's critical to eat a variety of healthful whole foods that are high in the vitamins and minerals listed below.

Because **B-complex vitamins** are water soluble and eliminated from the body through urination, they must be consumed on a regular basis. Vitamins B6 and B12 are essential for fertilization and hormonal function. **Fortified cereals, fortified soy-based meat substitutes, baked potatoes with skin, bananas, light-meat chicken and turkey, eggs, and spinach** are high in B6, whereas **beef, clams, mussels,**

crabs, salmon, poultry, soybeans, and fortified meals are high in B12.

Folic acid, often known as folate, is essential for the formation of genetic material in conjunction with vitamin B12. Folic Acid cannot be stored by the body and must be supplied on a regular basis. **Dark green leafy vegetables, apricots, avocados, carrots, egg yolks, liver, melons, whole grains, and yeast** are all natural sources.

Zinc is a necessary component of genetic material and plays an important role in male and female fertility (affecting sperm count). Because zinc is needed for normal cell division, adequate zinc levels are necessary during pregnancy. Natural sources of zinc include **oats, rye, almonds, pumpkin seeds, and peas.**

Essential Fatty Acids (EFAs) have an impact on every system in the body and are required for hormone synthesis to be balanced. EFAs can help women who have suffered many miscarriages by preventing blood clots from forming incorrectly (if clotting was an issue). They're mostly found in **fish oils.**

Vitamin E is a powerful antioxidant. In both men and women, low vitamin E levels can lead to infertility. **Wheat germ cereal, sunflower seeds, dark green leafy vegetables, nuts, brown grains, eggs, milk, organ meats, soy beans, and sweet potatoes** all contain this nutrient.

Vitamin C is an antioxidant that supports sperm production and may aid with ovulation health. Several systems in the human body require vitamin C to function properly and healthily. **Blackcurrants, raw red peppers, guavas, and citrus fruits such as oranges and grapefruits** are all high in vitamin C. **Strawberries, kiwifruit, broccoli, and Brussels sprouts** are also high in vitamin C.

Iron aids in the production of red blood cells and the transfer of oxygen throughout our bodies. Periods, childbirth, and blood loss can all lead to iron deficiency in the body (including blood donation). **Leafy green vegetables, beans, seafood, red meat, chicken, and soy** products are all high in iron.

Vitamin A is an antioxidant that the growing embryo requires throughout pregnancy. Natural sources include **carrots, tomatoes, cabbage, and spinach.**

27. Excellent Acne-Removal Methods

Most acne sufferers try to treat their irritated skin using topical face washes, soaps, lotions, and treatments. The best strategy to treat acne, however, is to change your diet and avoid acne-causing components like fried meals.

The first tip for treating acne is to consume a healthy diet rich in natural whole foods such as vegetables, fruits, whole grains, and beans. Trans-fatty acid-containing foods, such as milk and milk products, margarine, shortening, and other synthetically hydrogenated fats, as well as fried foods, should be avoided.

The prevalence of acne appears to be incorporated into the usual American diet. Americans consume a lot of food, which is frequently prepared in the most dangerous fats and oils. Not all fats are unhealthy, but the fats that most Americans consume, such as those found in ice cream, cheese, bacon, and milk, make people more prone to developing skin problems.

Acne cannot be effectively treated with creams and washes since the source of the problem is beneath the skin. Pimples and blemishes are produced by and other irritants lodged beneath the skin's oil glands and hair follicles, which are often caused by poor hygiene and a bad diet - such as a diet high in processed, greasy, fried, and sugary meals.

A skin-healthy diet includes raw and **gently cooked vegetables**, particularly Fiber-rich green leafy vegetables. Green veggies, especially fresh ones, are necessary. Include lean protein sources in your diet as well, such as r**ice, whole-grain bread, and potatoes**. These Fiber-rich meals aid in the maintenance of a healthy gastrointestinal tract, which is especially helpful in the treatment of acne.

Eat three healthful meals per day to get critical nutrients and to curb your cravings for sweets or greasy fried foods.

Acne can be reduced by eating foods strong in vitamin

A, such as **apricots, watermelon, and broccoli**, as well as zinc-rich foods like **lean beef, nuts, beans, and whole grains**. Drinking enough of water is also important for flushing out the toxins that trigger breakouts.

28. Flatulence-Relieving Foods

Flatulence can be caused by a variety of factors, including overeating, eating too rapidly, consuming too many refined carbs or artificial sweeteners, food allergies and intolerance, a vitamin B deficiency, excessive alcohol use, emotional stress, and parasites.

Lactose, which is present in dairy products such as milk and cheese, is one of the most common causes. Many other healthy foods, such as cabbage, beans, broccoli, Brussels sprouts, onions, cauliflower, whole wheat flour, radishes, bananas, and apricots, can also produce flatulence. Fortunately, by making a few changes to our dietary choices and eating habits, we can reduce or eliminate our risks of contracting this unpleasant disease.

Avoid overeating and chew your food slowly. Determine whether a certain food is causing the problem and eliminate it from your diet. After meals, chew a sprig of parsley. With your dinner, try lemon juice or apple cider vinegar in water. You might also try sipping your drinks gently with a straw to reduce the amount of air you take in while drinking.

Vitamin B complex, especially B3 (niacin) rich foods including **light-meat chicken, tuna, salmon, turkey, enriched wheat, peanuts, and fortified cereals**, can be useful since they aid in digestion and the conversion of food to energy.

Yogurts with acidophilus and peppermint oil in water, drunk with a meal, can also aid digestion. If the problem persists, you may want to try eating proteins and carbohydrates at different times of the day.

In addition, **peppermint and fennel-based teas** can help with occasional indigestion, especially if there is gas and a feeling of fullness. Ginger has been demonstrated to increase the flow of digestive juices, which is a natural mechanism that helps the digestive system.

<u>29. Foods That Fights The Herpes Virus</u>

Herpes outbreaks can be humiliating, as well as inconvenient and painful. And, in some cases, prescribed medication is ineffective in preventing flare-ups. However, with some thought and imagination, we may incorporate nutrients into our diet that will assist our bodies in fighting the herpes virus.

According to new research, cranberries may aid in the fight against herpes virus infection, which is one of the most frequent viral diseases in people.

Cranberries are already known to help prevent urinary tract infections by reducing the ability of certain E. coli bacteria to adhere to the urinary tract walls, and new research suggests that cranberries can also help suppress herpes type 2 by preventing the virus from attaching to and penetrating the walls. Cold sores and genital herpes are caused by HSV-2, or herpes simplex infection.

Broccoli protects against cancer, heart disease, and other major diseases. It contains a lot of vitamin C, which helps to boost the immune system. Broccoli may help decrease the replication of the herpes simplex virus.

Kelp is a fantastic, nutrient-dense marine vegetable that can also aid in the elimination of herpes outbreaks. It's also known as Laminaria, and it's a blood purifier.

Foods high in vitamins B, C, and E, as well as lysine, an amino acid, can also help improve the body's immune system to combat the herpes simplex virus. These are abundant in fish, bean sprouts, fruits, vegetables, and whole grain complex carbs.

Avoid processed sweets, stimulants like caffeine, alcohol, excessive sun exposure, and smoking, as these can all drain energy levels, compromising your immunity and ability to fight illnesses.

Stress is a key cause of herpes breakouts, so do everything you can to reduce stress in your life, including getting plenty of sleep, taking time to relax, getting lots of fresh air, and exercising.

30. Hives Relief Foods

Hives, also known as urticaria, are characterized by elevated white or yellow, itchy wheals surrounded by a red inflammatory region. It is a skin allergy that causes the body to release histamine into the affected tissues. The size of the wheal varies, with the larger ones occasionally coming together to form an uneven rash. They normally cause severe itchiness and develop on the limbs and trunk, but they can appear everywhere.

Acute urticaria develops quickly and usually lasts only a few hours; it is distinguished by a hot, faint feeling, and, on rare occasions, nausea. Chronic urticaria can last for an extended amount of time.

Drugs such as aspirin and penicillin are common triggers, as are dietary additives, food sensitivity such as milk, eggs, shellfish, and nuts, environmental factors such as exposure to cold, heat, or exposure to sunshine, tension and anxiety, as well as bites and stings

Vitamin C is present in all fruits and vegetables in some form. **Green peppers, citrus fruits and juices, strawberries, tomatoes, broccoli, turnip greens and other leafy greens, sweet and white potatoes, cantaloupe, and spinach are among the foods with the highest concentrations of vitamin C.** Vitamin C aids in the maintenance of a healthy immune system and the production of antihistamines. Green tea has also been linked to antihistamine properties.

Vitamin B12 has been demonstrated to reduce the severity and frequency of chronic outbreaks as well as the intensity of acute hives. Animal foods, fortified foods, and some fermented foods contain vitamin B12. Eggs, chicken, fish, dairy products, and soy products are all good sources of B12. Salmon and low-fat milk are particularly high in this nutrient.

If you have food allergies, you should keep a detailed dietary diary. Take note of what you ate when you had hives outbreaks, since it may be as simple as eliminating an item or several foods from your diet to avoid hives.

31. The Food That Prevents Bladder Infections

Cranberries may aid in the treatment of urinary tract infections (UTIs). They inhibit the ability of certain E. coli bacteria to attach to and permeate the bladder walls.

The E. coli that causes UTIs has distinctive small hairy points called fimbriae in around half of the cases. The bacteria attach themselves to the bladder via their fimbriae in order to grow and produce an infection. This is where cranberries, which contain a class of compounds known as Pro-anthocyanidins, come in.

They bind to the fimbriae of E. coli and impede their ability to adhere to the bladder walls. As a result, instead of producing an infection, the E. coli is flushed out in the urine. And because cranberries eliminate bacteria rather than killing them, E. coli is less likely to grow resistant.

It is critical that patients who are prone to UTIs consume cranberries or drink cranberry juice on a daily basis, since once the bacteria attach to the wall, the illness sets in, and cranberries can't assist. If you are prone, it is usually preferable to use cranberry products twice a day, as the effects of the cranberries wear off after around 10 hours.

You should also drink plenty of fluids on a regular basis to clear the bladder. Citrus fruits and vegetables strong in vitamin C are especially beneficial since they help increase the body's immunity and germ-fighting powers. Coffee, tea, and other caffeinated beverages, as well as alcohol, should be avoided.

Make sure to supplement your diet with plenty of vitamin B-rich foods, such as fortified cereals, lean meats, asparagus, almonds, and bananas, as they all aid the body in the digestion process and turning food to energy, which your body will want if it is fighting a UTI.

32. Food Poisoning Recovery Foods

Food poisoning is a broad phrase that encompasses the eating of tainted food, stomach flu, stress, drug interactions, nutrient deficiencies, or their excess. It can occur suddenly after eating; diarrhea or vomiting can occur 30 minutes to one hour after consuming chemically dangerous foods; within one to 12 hours of bacterial poisoning; and within 12 to 48 hours of viral or salmonella poisoning.

Food poisoning can be dangerous, and a medical expert should be notified immediately if there is trouble swallowing, speaking, or breathing; if there is a fever exceeding 100 degrees F; if the person can't even hold down drinks; or if there is severe diarrhea lasting more than two days.

The best treatment is to stop eating until all of the symptoms have gone away and the poisons have had a chance to leave your system. Drink plenty of fluids - vitamin C, **blackberry and peppermint teas** can be taken to strengthen the stomach, as can acidophilus-containing yoghurt to recolonize the lost bacteria in the intestine.

To restore the body's lost fluids and electrolytes, diluted sweetened drinks can be ingested, and the **BRAT diet (bananas, apples, rice, and toast)** can also be beneficial in getting the toxins out of the body.

Great care should be exercised when preparing dishes to avoid food poisoning. Avoid handling meals excessively, and when in question, throw it out – don't take a chance with leftovers if you're not sure how long they've been in your refrigerator.

Mint, lemon, raspberry, chamomile, or teas may also be beneficial in relieving stomach pain caused by food illness or stomach cramping. Ginger tea is also useful for soothing an upset stomach and promoting proper digestion.

Food poisoning can be a taxing and nutrient-depleting chore for your body, so try to get plenty of rest. Once you're feeling better, be sure to consume a well-balanced nutritious diet rich in iron, zinc, and vitamin

C to assist your body go back to normal.

<u>33. Foods That Can Help with Gout Symptoms</u>

Gout, also known as gouty arthritis, is caused by an excess of uric acid in the blood. The condition usually manifests itself in middle age and especially in men. It might be inherited or subsequent to another illness condition. The main sign of gout is severe joint pain and swelling, but gout normally affects one joint at a time and then may shift from one joint to another.

The kidneys remove uric acid from the body. However, in the case of gout, the body produces too much uric acid or the kidneys fail to work effectively, allowing the uric acid to build up in the joints in the form of uric acid crystals. This illness is excruciatingly uncomfortable. The build-up of these crystals in the joint produces considerable pain and swelling. The big toe joint is a common site for gout. Gout, on the other hand, can affect the ankle, knee, elbow, wrist, or finger.

Typically, the start is at night and is accompanied by intense pain, Edema, and inflammation. Rich foods and alcohol may contribute to an increase in uric acid and the severity of the symptoms. Fortunately, there are certain items that are likely already a part of your daily diet that can help relieve the symptoms of gout.

Apple's pectin and vitamin C content can help with gout relief. The vitamin C boosts the immune system, while the pectin keeps the joints flexible.

Onions are a potent antibacterial that protects the cardiovascular system. They are beneficial for urinary infections, and their diuretic activity aids in the treatment of arthritis, rheumatism, and gout.

Beets are higher in iron and other minerals than spinach, and the greens can assist with gout because the iron helps oxygenate and purify the bloodstream.

Drinking enough of water is also vital for keeping the kidneys filtering efficiently and preventing the creation of kidney stones. Purine-rich foods should be avoided because they account for around half of the uric acid produced in the body.

Purines are abundant in organ meats such as **liver, sweetbreads, brains, kidney, meat gravies, meat extracts, scallops, wild game, mackerel, herring, anchovies and sardines, and cauliflower.**

34. Foods for a Healthy Pregnancy

Pregnancy is an exciting moment in your life. It can also be physically, mentally, and spiritually stressful and exhausting at times. However, by nourishing your body with these fantastic foods, you'll be invigorated, strong, and sharp, and ready to greet your upcoming bundle of joy in a healthy and happy manner.

Protein, fiber, calcium, iron, thiamine, and niacin are all found in beans and legumes. When you have time, make a large batch of beans and freeze them in tiny containers. Canning types should be avoided because they are typically higher in sodium and have a reduced nutritional value due to the high temperatures used in processing.

Soybeans contain more protein than any other bean or legume, making them a must-have for both vegans and non-vegans. Soybeans include a variety of minerals, including calcium and iron.

Whole grains, such as brown rice, quinoa, millet, and oats, are high in fiber, minerals, protein, and B complex vitamins. Purchase the least processed grain kinds you can find, as many commercially prepared grains have had the nutritionally and nutritionally important germ and bran removed.

Dark green leafy vegetables, such as kale, collard greens, watercress, and spinach, are especially beneficial while pregnant or nursing because they contain a high concentration of vitamins and minerals, such as vitamins A and C, calcium, and iron. Dark leafy green veggies are also high in phytochemicals like beta carotene and lutein, which help to fight against cancer.

Cabbage family vegetables, such as broccoli, Brussels sprouts, and cabbage, are high in vitamin A, vitamin C, and calcium. They're also high in phytochemicals with anticancer effects. Dark green leafy vegetables and vegetables from the cabbage family include crucial elements that encourage a plentiful milk supply for your infant.

Nuts and seeds provide fiber, protein, minerals, and vital fatty acids. Consume flaxseeds, pumpkin seeds, almonds, and walnuts to acquire omega-3 fatty acids, which are essential for the development of your baby's brain and neurological system as well as your own health.

Nuts and seeds can be eaten raw or toasted, and they go well with dark leafy green vegetable salads.

Finally, it's critical to drink enough water and get plenty of rest throughout this period. A well-hydrated, well-rested body recovers faster and is better prepared to face the obstacles that life with a new born baby presents.

35. Providing Nutritional Hope to Schizophrenic Patients

Schizophrenia is a challenging disease to identify and treat. It is defined as any of a series of psychotic disorders characterized by detachment from reality, illogical patterns of thought, delusions, and hallucinations, as well as other emotional, behavioral, or intellectual abnormalities to varied degrees.

Recent research reveals that patients suffering from schizophrenia may benefit from increasing their intake of B3 (niacin), essential fatty acids (EFAs), and whole grain carbs to help level out blood sugar levels and reduce episodes of hypoglycemia.

Light-meat chicken, tuna, salmon, and turkey are examples of niacin-rich foods, as are enriched flour, peanuts, and fortified cereals. Niacin is essential for digestion and the conversion of food into energy. As a result, it also plays a role in the critical fatty acid metabolism of the brain, which is disrupted in schizophrenia.

Because these mechanisms in the brain are interrupted, essential fatty acids must be a staple in the diet of a schizophrenia patient. They must be taken through food because they cannot be produced by the body. EFAs can be found in fish, shellfish, flaxseed, pumpkin seeds, dark green leafy vegetables, and walnuts.

Essential fatty acids are involved in numerous metabolic processes, and there is evidence that insufficient amounts of essential fatty acids, or the incorrect balance of essential fatty acid types, may be a cause in a variety of disorders, including schizophrenia.

Some schizophrenia patients experience spells of hypoglycemia, which can be substantially alleviated by eating nutritious, whole grain carbs like whole grain breads and pastas, which assist the body maintain a constant blood glucose level.

Other research indicates that some schizophrenia patients have food allergies, which have a significant impact on their thinking and behavior. As a result, keeping a detailed food log and paying close attention to moods and thought patterns after eating are essential.

According to research, some schizophrenia patients have high levels of copper, a necessary metallic element that can harm the brain in large doses. Vitamin B6, found in **bananas, turkey, and spinach,** and zinc, found in **red meats, peanuts, chickpeas, and almonds,** can both assist the body eliminate excess copper.

36. Sinusitis-Relieving foods

Sinusitis is just inflammation of the sinuses, but this offers little clue of the suffering and pain that this ailment may inflict. Chronic sinusitis, defined as sinusitis that lasts at least three weeks, affects an estimated 32 million people in the United States, and Americans spend millions of dollars each year on drugs that promise sinus relief.

Sinusitis symptoms include fever, fatigue, and exhaustion, as well as a cough that may be more acute at night and a runny nose or nasal congestion. Furthermore, mucus leakage from the sinuses down the back of the throat (postnasal drip) can create a painful throat. However, by incorporating a few foods from specific vitamin groups, we can reduce our chances of becoming plagued with this unpleasant and inconvenient disease.

Citrus fruits, red berries, tomatoes, potatoes, broccoli, cauliflower, Brussels sprouts, red and green bell peppers, cabbage, and spinach are all high in vitamin C, which aids in immune system health.

The B-complex vitamins are a set of eight vitamins that include thiamine (B1), riboflavin (B2), niacin (B3), and folic acid (B9) and are required for a healthy neurological system, carbohydrate processing for energy, and red blood cell formation. **Organ meats, beans, whole grain cereals, oatmeal, potatoes, salmon, bananas, and spinach** are just a few of the numerous vitamin B food members with high quantities of this nutrient.

Vitamin E is found in a variety of foods, including vegetable oils, almonds, green leafy vegetables, and fortified cereals. Vitamin E is an antioxidant that protects your cells from the impacts of free radicals, which are potentially harmful by products of energy metabolism. Free radicals can cause cell damage and may play a role in the development of cardiovascular disease and cancer. Vitamin E has also been found to help with immunological function.

Inhaling steam from a vaporizer or a hot cup of water can help to relieve sinusitis. Saline nasal spray, which may be acquired at a drugstore, is another option. A hot water bottle, hot, wet compresses, or an electric heating pad applied to the inflamed area can also provide relief.

95

A person who is prone to sinus problems, especially if they are allergic, should avoid cigarette smoke and other air pollution. Allergies create nasal inflammation, which predisposes a patient to a severe reaction to any allergen. The nasal-sinus membranes thicken as a result of alcohol use. Avoid dairy items since they cause your body to generate more mucus.

37. Foods for Beautiful Skin

It's been stated that we are what we eat, and this is certainly true when it comes to our skin. It's our largest organ, and it deserves all the dietary attention we can offer it. So, think about what you've been feeding yourself, and hence your skin.

Vitamin A is one of the most important components of skin health, and low-fat dairy products are one of the greatest sources of it. Our skin's health is thought to be dependent on vitamin A. **Low-fat yoghurt** is high in not only vitamin A, but also acidophilus, the "living" bacteria that is beneficial to intestinal health. It turns out that it may also have an effect on the skin since it promotes digestion. Cod liver oil, sweet potatoes, carrots, green vegetables, and fortified breakfast cereals are also rich sources of vitamin A.

It's also crucial to consume antioxidant-rich foods like **blackberries, blues, strawberries,** and **plums**. The advantages of these foods for healthy skin are numerous. These fruits' antioxidants and other phytochemicals can protect skin cells, reducing the risk of harm. This, in turn, protects against premature ageing and keeps skin looking younger for a longer period of time. Other antioxidant-rich fruits and vegetables include **artichokes, black, red, and pinto beans, prunes,** and **nuts.**

Essential fatty acids (EFAs) are necessary for healthy skin. Salmon, walnuts, canola oil, and flax seed are all good additions. EFAs maintain the health of cell membranes and allow nutrients to pass through.

We also require healthy oils that include more than just vital fatty acids. Eating high-quality oils keeps skin lubricated and makes it look and feel healthier overall. Look for cold-pressed oils, such as olive or extra virgin oil. We only need approximately two teaspoons of healthy oils every day, so utilize them judiciously.

Selenium is essential for the health of skin cells. For this essential nutrient, eat **whole-wheat bread, muffins,** and **cereals**, as well as **turkey, tuna, and Brazil nuts.** According to recent research, if selenium levels are high, even sun-damaged skin may suffer minimal, if any, damage.

Choosing whole grain complex carbohydrates has been shown to have a substantial effect on insulin levels. Processed and processed sugars can promote inflammation, which can lead to acne breakouts.

Green tea has anti-inflammatory effects and preserves the cell membrane. It may potentially aid in the prevention or reduction of skin cancer risks.

Water is vital to your general health, and it also has a significant impact on the quality of your skin. Skin that is well-hydrated seems healthy and youthful. It also aids in the removal of poisons from your system, reducing their ability to cause harm.

38. Foods for Chronic Fatigue Syndrome Relief

The primary symptoms of chronic fatigue syndrome (CFS) are generalized physical and mental exhaustion. Tiredness can be caused by a variety of factors. Just because you're tired all the time doesn't mean you have CFS. The problem must last for at least six months and be accompanied by other symptoms such as memory loss, sore throat, headaches, and muscle/joint discomfort without swelling or redness.

Though there are multiple potential causes of CFS, inadequate nutrition is the root cause of all fatigue. Other possible factors include poor digestion, food allergies, obesity, sleep issues, tension, or depression. Cigarette smoking, alcohol, and drug use are all risk factors.

Physical and mental exhaustion are the most common symptoms. It can be severe enough that people are unable to fully participate in typical, everyday activities. Even having plenty of rest does not appear to make a difference for the majority of sufferers.

However, by making simple lifestyle adjustments and eating a diet rich in whole food nutrients, almost anyone may help prevent or even reverse these symptoms.

You can eat a more nutritious diet that includes primarily fresh **fruits, vegetables,** and **whole grains. Citrus fruits, berries, tomatoes, potatoes, broccoli, cauliflower, Brussels sprouts, red and green bell peppers, cabbage,** and **spinach** are all high in vitamin C, which aids in immune system health. Zinc has the same effect. Zinc is found in a variety of foods, including **red meat, fortified cereals, peanuts,** and **dairy products.**

Focus on **fish** high in omega-3 oils and lean poultry for protein since they are high in essential fatty acids (EFAs), which help promote circulation and oxygen uptake with adequate red blood cell elasticity and function. EFAs must be obtained through diet because the body cannot produce them. EFA deficiency has been linked to decreased mental capacity and immunological function.

Other things that will assist include reducing stress, obtaining plenty of excellent quality rest, and engaging in frequent moderate exercise. Drink plenty of fresh, clean water and avoid sweets, coffee, sodas, processed foods, and salty foods. Set attainable goals and believe positively.

<u>39. Foods To Improve Your Circulatory System</u>

Circulation issues can manifest themselves in a variety of ways. Some symptoms include weariness as a result of impaired vascular function, which can lead to additional symptoms like dizziness and fainting.

Inability to concentrate, coldness in the hands or feet, headaches, angina, and elevated blood pressure are all symptoms that the circulatory system is malfunctioning. There are nutrient-dense foods that we may integrate into our meals to guarantee that our circulatory system is functioning optimally.

If your circulation is weak, it is critical that you maintain your vitamin C levels, since this will assist to avoid artery hardening and arterial ballooning. **Citrus fruits, red berries, tomatoes, potatoes, broccoli, cauliflower, Brussels sprouts, red and green bell peppers, cabbage,** and **spinach** are all excellent sources of vitamin C, which promotes a healthy immune system and is required to help make collagen, which holds cells together and is essential in maintaining the integrity and strength of the arteries and veins.

Leafy green vegetables, almonds, hazelnuts, and **vegetable oils** such as **sunflower, canola, and soybean** are all high in antioxidants, which are well known for their potential to protect against diseases such as cancer and heart disease. **Broccoli, cabbage,** and **kale** are other excellent suppliers.

Nuts are high in healthy, unsaturated fatty acids, and studies demonstrate a link between nut consumption and a lower risk of ischemic heart disease. These essential fatty acids are abundant in walnuts, pecans, and hazelnuts.

Fish oils, such as those found in sardines, may aid in the treatment or prevention of atherosclerosis, angina, heart attack, congestive heart failure, arrhythmias, stroke, and peripheral vascular disease. Fish oils aid to preserve arterial wall flexibility, prevent blood clotting, lower blood pressure, and normalize heart rhythm.

Vitamin E is an antioxidant that shields bodily tissue

from the harmful effects of unstable molecules known as free radicals. Free radicals can cause harm to cells, tissues, and organs by damaging the cell walls of arteries in the circulatory system. Vitamin E is also necessary for the production of red blood cells. Wheat germ, corn, almonds, seeds, olives, spinach, and asparagus are all high in vitamin E.

40. Foods to Fight Liver Cirrhosis

Cirrhosis is the replacement of injured liver cells with fibrous scar tissue, which affects the liver's vital processes. Cirrhosis is caused by excessive alcohol use (the most prevalent cause), common viral hepatitis, bile duct obstruction, and exposure to certain medicines or toxic substances.

Cirrhotic patients frequently experience loss of appetite, nausea, vomiting, and weight loss, giving them an emaciated appearance. The development of this liver disease is not caused solely by diet. People who are well-nourished but use a lot of alcohol, for example, are predisposed to alcoholic disease.

Cirrhotic adults require a protein-rich diet in order for their liver cells to repair. However, too much protein increases the quantity of ammonia in the blood, whereas too little protein reduces liver repair. Doctors must carefully prescribe the appropriate dosage of protein for cirrhotic patients.

A balanced diet with appropriate calories, lipids, and carbohydrates, in addition to protein, can actually help the injured liver create new liver cells. In reality, in some cases of liver illness, diet becomes a necessary type of treatment.

Grains and legumes are excellent sources of protein for those with cirrhosis. Red meat should be avoided since the liver is not functioning optimally and will most likely have difficulty digesting fats. Low-fat protein can also be found in **nuts, seeds,** and **soy** products.

Oatmeal, brown rice, whole grain breads, and **pastas** should all be included in a healthy balanced diet since they are all whole grain carbs that provide a consistent flow of energy, which is necessary for your body's ability to heal.

B-complex vitamins are found in cereals, breads, potatoes, and legumes, and they assist to boost metabolism, maintain healthy skin and muscle tone, improve immunological and neurological system function, and promote cell development and division —

including that of red blood cells, which helps avoid anemia. They also work together to treat the symptoms and causes of, which is crucial to bear in mind when nursing your body back to health.

Citrus fruits, red berries, tomatoes, potatoes, broccoli, cauliflower, brussels sprouts, red and green bell peppers, cabbage, and spinach are all high in vitamin C, which aids in immune system health. It is critical to maintain as much health as possible during the healing process so that your body can focus on liver repair.

A well-balanced nutrition plan and a strong, proactive connection with your healthcare practitioner, together with plenty of rest and plenty of fresh water to help flush the toxins from your system, should put you well on the road to recovery.

<u>41. Foods That Make You Move</u>

It's no surprise that so many Americans suffer from constipation. Our meat-and-processed-food diet is deficient in fiber. Most of us are lucky if we obtain half of the recommended 30 grams of fiber per day. Without that mass in our diet, bowel movements can become nearly intractable.

The human digestive tract was intended to process unprocessed plant meals high in dietary fiber, such as beans, leafy greens, fresh and dried fruits and vegetables, and whole grains. Dietary fiber intake increases both the frequency and quantity of bowel movements, reducing stool transit time and the absorption of toxins from the stool.

Consume eight to twelve **8-ounce glasses of pure water every day**. Hard, dry stools are a common symptom of dehydration. A decent rule of thumb is to drink a glass of water as soon as you wake up and then every hour thereafter.

Try incorporating wheat or barley grass into your everyday routine. Mix two to three teaspoons of a nutrient-rich blend of dried wheat and/or barley grass with water, and repeat later in the day. These drinks have a healing effect on the digestive tract and are especially beneficial for constipation.

Bran and prunes are particularly useful in alleviating constipation as a supplement to a healthy, high-fiber diet. Prunes, both whole and juiced, have laxative properties. A dose of eight ounces is generally sufficient. A comparable amount of aloe vera juice is also beneficial.

Vitamin C-rich meals can also help with food and nutrient absorption. Vitamin C-rich foods include **parsley, broccoli, bell pepper, strawberries, oranges, lemon juice, papaya, cauliflower, kale, mustard greens, and Brussels sprouts.**

42. Superb Crohn's Disease Treatments

When the small intestine gets inflamed, as it frequently does with Crohn's disease, the gut becomes less able to digest and absorb nutrients from meals. Such nutrients, as well as unabsorbed bile salts, can escape to variable degrees into the large intestine depending on how severely the small intestine has been injured by inflammation. This is one of the causes of malnutrition in Crohn's disease patients, in addition to a lack of appetite.

Furthermore, even if the colon is not injured, partially digested foods that pass through the large intestine interfere with water conservation. As a result, when Crohn's disease attacks the small intestine, it can cause diarrhea as well as malnutrition. If the large intestine is also irritated, the diarrhea may grow worse.

People with Crohn's disease who have an affected small intestine are more likely to become malnourished due to loss of appetite, poor digestion, and malabsorption, as well as the fact that a chronic disease like Crohn's tends to increase the caloric needs of the body due to the energy the body consumes during a flare-up.

One of the ways the body recovers and heals itself is through proper eating. As a result, all efforts must be done to prevent malnutrition. Protein is an important nutrient in the recovery process. Consume lean cuts of chicken and fish as sources of protein. Protein deficit can cause fatigue, insulin resistance, and muscle mass loss.

Iron deficiency is frequent in patients with ulcerative colitis and Crohn's disease, although it is less common in people with small intestinal illness. It is caused by blood loss as a result of colon inflammation and ulceration.

Combine iron-rich foods like **poultry, soy foods**, and some fortified foods like **whole grain cereals** with vitamin C-rich fruits and vegetables including **potatoes, broccoli, cauliflower, Brussels sprouts, red and green bell peppers, and cabbage.** This dietary combination enhances iron absorption, while vitamin C boosts the immune system.

Limit your intake of high-fiber foods such as nuts, seeds, and corn. High-fiber diets also produce contractions in the large intestine, which can result in cramping. They may also cause diarrhea because the small intestine does not digest them entirely. A low-fiber diet is sometimes required to reduce stomach pain and cramping symptoms.

It may also be important to supplement your diet with nutritional supplements to ensure that your body receives the appropriate vitamins and minerals.

43. Foods For A Healthy Thyroid

Thyroid disease affects an estimated 27 million Americans, with more than half going misdiagnosed. Thyroid disease affects practically every aspect of health and is frequently misunderstood. It is also far too often neglected and misdiagnosed. Taking care of it through proper nutrition is a wise move in the correct way. Here are several foods that research has shown can promote thyroid health, as well as some to avoid.

Coconut and **coconut butter**, also known as coconut oil, have been used as a food and medicinal from the beginning of time. Unlike saturated animal fats found in meats and dairy items, coconut butter is a raw saturated fat that contains fatty acids that the body can easily digest and convert to energy. It also helps to regulate thyroid function, according to research.

Kelp is a fantastic, nutrient-rich sea vegetable. It also goes by the name Laminaria and contains a natural ingredient that enhances flavour and tenderizes. Kelp acts as a blood purifier and promotes the health of the adrenal, pituitary, and thyroid glands. Its natural iodine content may aid in the normalization of thyroid-related illnesses such as obesity and lymph system congestion.

Turkey is high in lean protein and low in calories, making it a great healthy meal option. Turkey also includes selenium, which has been shown to reduce cancer formation, boost the immune system, and aid in thyroid hormone metabolism.

Thyroid sufferers should avoid consuming goitrogens, which are drugs that decrease thyroid gland activity and can also promote thyroid hypertrophy. Foods containing goitrogens include broccoli, cauliflower, Brussels sprouts, cabbage, mustard, kale, turnips, and canola oil. Soy and peanuts contain goitrogens as well and should be avoided.

Because copper and iron are so critical for thyroid function, thyroid patients should take the effort to ensure they obtain enough of them in their diets. Copper-rich foods include organ meats, clams, crabs, cashews, sunflower seeds, wheat bran cereals, whole-grain products, oysters and cocoa products.

Iron-rich foods include leafy **green vegetables, beans, seafood, red meat,** and **chicken**. To help increase your body's iron absorption efficiency, supplement your iron consumption with enough levels of vitamin C from foods such as **citrus fruits, red berries, tomatoes, potatoes,** and **bell peppers.**

44. Juices

Juice is a natural water supply that feeds the body with protein, carbs, vital fatty acids, vitamins, and minerals that are quickly and efficiently absorbed. Fresh juice is also high in enzymes and colours including carotenes, chlorophyll, and flavonoids.

Juicing fresh fruits and vegetables gives several nutritional benefits that are critical for weight loss. Furthermore, diets high in raw foods are strongly connected with weight loss, improved blood sugar control, and lower blood pressure.

A raw food diet is more filling for your appetite. Cooking can destroy up to 97 percent of the water-soluble vitamins A, D, E, and K. Because uncooked foods, such as juices, have more vitamins and nutrients, they are more fulfilling to the body, preventing it from feeling deprived of nutrition. This means that your metabolism will continue to function properly and your weight loss efforts will be successful.

Juicing jump-starts your body's digestive process and allows for rapid absorption of high-quality nourishment, which can lead to greater energy. This is one of the many advantages of **losing weight** through better eating. Fresh juices, when combined with a well-balanced diet, will provide you the energy you need to burn more calories, fat, and provide the fuel you need for physical exercise.

Juicing, on the other hand, removes the fiber from these nutrient-dense foods. As a result, make sure to incorporate a sufficient number of fiber-rich foods in your regular diet. Juicing should be used as a supplement to a well-balanced healthy diet, not as a replacement.

So, with a little forethought and ingenuity, juicing could complement your well-balanced diet and add some spice to it. The internet is a terrific resource for juicing recipes and information, and as more people realize the benefits of raw foods and juicing, books and magazine articles promote the benefits and offer recipe suggestions.

45. Organic Foods Are Associated with Better Health

Organic food contains no genetically modified organisms, is farmed without the use of artificial pesticides and fertilizers, and is derived from animals that were not routinely administered antibiotics, growth hormones, or other drugs. Organic goods, which were formerly exclusively available in small stores or farmers markets, are becoming much more broadly available.

Organic foods have been proven to boost your immune system, enhance your sleep, help you lose weight more easily, and improve your blood work, to name a few benefits. Organic food can have more intense, genuine flavours as well as a higher vitamin and mineral content.

And, while eating organic foods makes logical sense, some people are concerned about the cost. However, with careful planning and preparation, turning organic can be pretty economical. And the peace of mind that comes from knowing you and your family are eating foods that haven't been pesticide-treated or genetically modified is worth the extra money.

Pesticides used by conventional farmers can have a variety of detrimental effects on your health, including neurotoxicity, endocrine disruption, carcinogenicity, and immune system suppression. Pesticide exposure has also been associated with miscarriages in women and may alter male reproductive function.

Furthermore, conventional produce contains fewer nutrients than organic stuff. Conventional vegetables have only 83 percent of the nutrients found in organic produce. Organic crops include much higher quantities of minerals such as vitamin C, iron, magnesium, and phosphorus, as well as significantly lower levels of nitrates (a toxin).

So, for optimal health benefits, it's a good idea to buy and eat organic produce and free-range organic meals as often as possible.

Furthermore, knowing that you're helping to protect

the environment by avoiding harmful pesticides and chemicals that can result in topsoil loss, toxic runoff and resulting water pollution, soil contamination and poisoning, and the death of insects, birds, critters, and beneficial soil organisms should make you feel even better.

46. A Raw Foods Diet Is Good For Your Health

Lowering cholesterol and triglyceride levels, decreasing cravings, limiting overeating, emptying the body of accumulated toxins, balancing hormones, maintaining blood glucose levels, and curing degenerative diseases are just a few of the benefits recommended for following such a diet.

Raw diet adherents claim several health benefits, including greater energy levels, enhanced skin appearance, improved digestion, weight loss, and a lower risk of heart disease, to mention a few.

Proponents think that enzymes are a food's life power and that each dish includes its own unique blend. These enzymes aid in the thorough digestion of foods, eliminating the need for our bodies to manufacture their own cocktail of digestive enzymes.

When you initially begin a raw foods diet, you may

experience certain negative effects. Some detoxification effects may be felt as your body strives to rid itself of toxins. This may include headaches, nausea, and moderate depression on occasion. If these symptoms persist, you should seek the assistance of someone who is familiar with detoxification symptoms.

Following a raw food diet necessitates meticulous meal planning to ensure you get enough critical nutrients, vitamins, and minerals. In some cases, especially when first starting out, it may be prudent to consider taking nutritional supplements. If you don't already have them, you'll need to purchase some kitchen appliances to make the food.

Raw food preparation is simplified by the use of a sturdy juicer, a blender, and a large food processor. You should also consider acquiring large containers for soaking sprouts, grains, and beans, as well as storage. A long-lasting juice extractor for fruits and vegetables.

The best approach to start a raw foods lifestyle is to gradually transition into it. Begin by incorporating 70 to 80 percent raw foods into your diet. Consume fruit and salads throughout the day, and in the evening, have a cooked veggie dish with a salad. This should make the shift simpler on your body and, ideally, reduce the adverse effects of detoxification.

This is also an emotional moment, so give yourself plenty of time to make the transition. Keeping a journal while going through the process can be beneficial. You'll be experiencing the benefits of a healthy, detoxifying raw foods diet before you realize it.

47. The Hay Diet Treats A Chemical Condition In The Body

In 1911, Dr. William Howard Hay pioneered food mixing. His own health began to worsen after 16 years of medical practice, and he developed high blood pressure, Bright's disease (today more widely known as acute or chronic nephritis, a kidney disease), and a dilated heart.

Dr. Hay was inspired to cure his own problems because there was no medication for dilated hearts at the time. His main idea is that there is only one underlying source of health problems, and that is a chemical imbalance in the body.

He accomplished this by eating 'fundamentally,' as he put it, by consuming things in their natural form and avoiding combining proteins and grains at the same meal. The incorrect chemical condition is acidity, which is caused by the production and accumulation of acid from digestion and metabolic products in proportions greater than the body's ability to remove.

Dr. Hay recommended **fresh air, exercise, and general lifestyle improvements** in addition to nutritional changes. The basic rules of this diet are as follows:

- starches and sugar should not be eaten together with proteins and acid fruits at the same meal; vegetables, salads, and fruits should play a major role in the diet; proteins,
- starches, and fats should be consumed in small amounts, with only whole grain unprocessed starches being used; and finally,
- at least 4 hours should occur between different food groups' meals. It is often referred to as the "food mixing" diet. Acid foods, such as meat, fish, and dairy, are high in protein, whereas alkaline foods, such as rice, wheat, and potatoes, are high in carbs.

The Hay Diet's basic rules help reverse chronic and degenerative illnesses like constipation, indigestion, and arthritis. Asthmatics and allergy patients may benefit from it. It can also promote natural weight loss, lowering the health concerns associated with obesity, such as diabetes, gallstones, and coronary heart disease.

48. Water Is the Lifeblood of Our Bodies

Humans can go for weeks without food but only a few days without water. The human body is composed of around 55 to 75% water. Water is found in lean muscle, fat, and bones, as well as blood, digestive fluids, urine, and perspiration.

We require fresh amounts of water every day to compensate for losses through the lungs, skin, urine, and faeces since the body cannot store water. Water is required to maintain the health and integrity of all cells in the body, to keep the bloodstream liquid enough to flow through blood vessels, to help eliminate by products of the body's metabolism, to flush out toxins, to regulate body temperature through sweating, to lubricate and cushion joints, and to transport nutrients and oxygen to the body's cells, to name a few. Drinking refreshing, clean water helps to reduce the risk of some diseases.

The use of decaffeinated and alcoholic beverages significantly increases the loss of bodily water through urine. These beverages have a diuretic effect, which means they cause the kidneys to excrete more pee. We lose not only water, but also water-soluble vitamins like vitamin C, vitamin B (thiamine), and other B complex vitamins. You should drink one glass of clean water for every caffeinated or alcoholic beverage you consume.

A diet rich in **fruits and vegetables** will provide approximately **4 glasses** of water per day. Even with a diet high in fruits and vegetables, an additional **6 to 8 glasses of water per day** is required to deliver enough water to meet the body's daily demands. You should drink one glass of clean water for every caffeinated or alcoholic beverage you consume.

Dehydration happens when the body's water content is too low. This can be easily remedied by increasing fluid intake. Headaches, lethargy, mood swings, and delayed responses are all symptoms of dehydration, as are dry nasal passages, dry or cracked lips, dark-coloured urine, weakness, weariness, confusion, and hallucinations. Urination eventually stops, the kidneys fail, and the body is unable to eliminate poisonous waste materials. In extreme cases, this could result in death.

Each day, six to eight glasses of fluids of varying types can be drunk. Physically active persons, youngsters, people living in hot or humid climates, and breastfeeding mothers may require more than eight glasses. Sedentary people, the elderly, people living in cold climates, and people who consume a lot of high-water-content foods may require less water.

49. A Macrobiotic Diet Can Help You Maintain a Healthy Diet And Lifestyle

Macrobiotics adherents think that food, especially the quality of food, has a greater impact on our lives than is typically assumed. It is supposed to have an impact on our health, happiness, and well-being.

They emphasize moving away from processed meals and toward more natural and traditional food preparation methods. They argue that it is healthier for them and their families to eat less processed, more natural foods and employ more traditional methods of food preparation.

Macrobiotics, rather than scientific dietary advice, stress locally grown, organically grown whole grain cereals, legumes, vegetables, fruits, seaweed, and fermented soy products blended into meals according to the notion of balance between yin and yang qualities.

Macrobiotic diets are based on the concept of **Yin and Yang. Cereals, fruit, beans, nuts, and vegetables, as well as rice,** comprise the majority of the diet and are considered neutral and naturally balanced in terms of Yin and Yang.

Foods that are either exceedingly Yin or excessively Yang in nature are eaten infrequently, if at all. **Coffee, tropical fruit, sugar, soft dairy products, veggies, wine, and honey are all very Yin items. Poultry, meat, firm dairy products such as hard cheeses, and eggs are examples of Yang products.**

Natural, unprocessed foods, complex carbs, and vegetables are abundant in the macrobiotic diet. It is low in saturated fats while supplying necessary fats. Food should be cultivated naturally and consumed fresh. The Macrobiotic way of life also regulates how food is cooked. Rice should be cooked in a pressure cooker rather than a microwave. Food should be eaten and chewed slowly and calmly.

Low-fat, high-fiber diets are also thought to help against certain types of cancer. Furthermore, the macrobiotic emphasis on fresh, unprocessed foods may be useful to persons suffering from food allergies and chemical sensitivities.

Followers believe that the macrobiotic food and lifestyle, when balanced and harmonious, produce the finest possible circumstances for health. They believe that the diet has numerous favourable health advantages, including a general sense of well-being, and that certain studies show that people who follow the diet have a lower risk of heart disease and certain types of cancer.

<u>50. Essentials of a Healthful Diet</u>

According to the United States Department of Agriculture, a healthy diet emphasizes fruits, vegetables, whole grains, and fat-free or low-fat milk and milk products; includes lean meats, poultry, fish, eggs, beans and nuts; and is low in trans fats, saturated fats, cholesterol, salt (sodium), and added sugars. But which minerals and nutrients are essential for our health and well-being? When trying to increase your vitamin and mineral intake, consider these nutrient-dense meals.

Vitamin A is required for healthy vision and immune system function. Cod liver oil, dairy products, sweet potatoes, and dark green leafy vegetables are all excellent natural vitamin A sources.

Vitamin B1, often known as thiamine, is required for the body to digest carbohydrates. Thiamine is abundant in **whole grain breads, cereals, and pastas.**

Riboflavin, often known as vitamin B2, is found in **fortified cereals, almonds, asparagus, eggs, and beef.** It is involved in a variety of bodily activities, including the conversion of food into energy and the generation of red blood cells.

Niacin, often known as vitamin B3, is found in foods such as **lean chicken, tuna, salmon, and turkey, as well as enriched wheat, peanuts, and fortified cereals**. It promotes digestion and also plays an important function in the conversion of food into energy.

Vitamin B6 is found in **fortified cereals, fortified soy-based meat substitutes, baked potatoes with skin, bananas, light-meat chicken and turkey, eggs, and spinach.** It is essential for a healthy neurological system and aids in the breakdown of proteins and stored carbohydrates.

Vitamin B12 is necessary for the development of red blood cells and can be found in **beef, clams, mussels, crabs, salmon, poultry, and soybeans.**

Citrus fruits, red berries, tomatoes, potatoes, broccoli, cauliflower, Brussels sprouts, red and green bell peppers, cabbage, and spinach are all high in vitamin C, which is essential for immune system function and the production of chemical messengers in the brain.

Vitamin D can be found in **fortified milk, cheese, and cereals, as well as egg yolks and salmon**, but it can also be produced by the body through sun exposure. It is required for calcium processing and bone and tooth health.

Vitamin E is an antioxidant that is crucial for the health of your skin. To obtain this essential nutrient, consume enough of **leafy green vegetables, almonds, hazelnuts, and vegetable oils such as sunflower, canola, and soybean.**

ABOUT THE AUTHOR

"Henry H Steele, author of Self-Help: Best 101 Tips and Growing Your Self-Confidence: What You Need to Know, among other books, lives in Brooklyn, New York, with his wife and two children."